I0712078

BE KIND TO YOURSELF

THE SIMPLEST PATH TO YOUR WELL-BEING
BY UNDERSTANDING ITS BIOLOGY
AND FOLLOWING A FOUR-STEP PRACTICE

GHADA ABDELGAWAD, M.D.

BALBOA.PRESS

A DIVISION OF HAY HOUSE

Balboa Press books may be ordered through booksellers or by contacting:

Balboa Press
A Division of Hay House
1663 Liberty Drive
Bloomington, IN 47403
www.balboapress.com
844-682-1282

Print information available on the last page.

ISBN: 979-8-7652-5683-1 (sc)
ISBN: 979-8-7652-5684-8 (e)

Library of Congress Control Number: 2024922832

Balboa Press rev. date: 10/22/2024

I dedicate this book to my husband for loving and believing in me; my son, to whom the credit goes for writing this book; and my daughter, who is a continuous source of love and inspiration.

May you be well, happy, peaceful, and loved wherever you are .

CONTENTS

INTRODUCTION

WHY THIS BOOK?

I have been practicing psychiatry since 1997. I started as a resident, progressed to a specialist, and am currently a psychiatry consultant. As someone who has worked in this field for more than twenty-five years, I recognize that there is still a stigma around seeking psychiatric care. This can prevent many people from achieving the well-being they deserve.

There are no coincidences; everything happens for a reason. This book has found you for a reason. In this book, I will guide you to the well-being you deserve. You deserve it not for anything you did but simply because you were born blessed and worthy, and your life journey is to find your way back to this fact.

I strongly advocate for promoting the overall well-being of every individual, acknowledging that certain individuals may only require guidance while others may require more extensive interventions due to difficult circumstances.

This book aims to remind you of your inherent value as a human being. It's important to note that while I cannot solve your problems, I can offer guidance toward your personal journey of growth.

This journey is yours to embark on, and it has the potential to positively influence not only your own life but those around you. If you want to be the best parent, friend, partner, or colleague you can be, you must first take care of yourself.

Nobody can or should control your thinking or decisions. As my patients begin their journey toward healing, they commonly wish they had this knowledge earlier.

I chose to write the book as brief and simple as possible, minimizing the use of medical jargon to ensure it is easily applicable and practical to readers. To truly benefit from the valuable information contained within, I intentionally kept the book concise. It's crucial to incorporate it into your daily life, which will require revisiting the material multiple times.

The first chapter explains how your mind works. The second chapter will be about the scientific background of stress and how it affects every cell of your body. In the third chapter, I talk about some cases from my clinic that you may relate to or may help you understand yourself better. The fourth chapter offers practical exercises designed to guide you to your well-being.

The central message of this book is to be kind to yourself. You cannot achieve well-being or extend kindness to others without self-compassion first. This principle will be emphasized frequently as a constant reminder.

I totally believe in your well-being, not for anything you have done but because you are born blessed and worthy, and I hope I can guide you back to believing it.

May this book help you find the love, peace, joy, and well-being you deserve.

A GUIDE TO EFFECTIVELY UTILIZE THIS BOOK

As mentioned earlier, I wrote this book as concisely as possible for you to adapt the information to fit your daily life.

The first step is to read the book completely. Most of the information will flood you with a sense of relief. Some information will be new and interesting, and some will feel strange.

Read the book as many times as you feel necessary before trying to make any changes to your life.

Start your journey and try to read this book every time you feel any negative emotions.

May you be well, happy, peaceful, and loved wherever you are.

1

HOW OUR MINDS WORK

Your mind is valuable. It won't be an exaggeration to say it's your most precious possession. First, let's distinguish between the terms *mind* and *brain*. By mind, I refer to your thoughts, emotions, and perceptions. The brain is a vital physical organ that is well-protected inside your skull, emphasizing its significance. To simplify things, there are two levels of your mind, conscious and subconscious. The conscious mind refers to when you are attentive, analytical, and in the process of making a decision. Your subconscious mind is essentially a storage space where you keep your emotions, experiences, and beliefs. As an example of both: you need your conscious mind to learn how to drive, but after a while it becomes a subconscious process. You may drive home from work without thinking about it, especially if you take the same routes you are used to taking. But with any change—for example, a road closure—you will have to use your conscious mind to plan a different route. Whatever you think about actively is part of your conscious mind. Whatever you do without thinking is coming from your subconscious. We tend to adopt most subconscious mind programs in childhood, or unintentionally from culture, family, or our surroundings.

Remember that any mood you are in now—good or bad—is a result of your current thought pattern, coming mainly from your subconscious mind. You tend to act according to your programs without thinking, considering your behavior and perception as normal, expected, or even worse, not under your control. How many times did you hear yourself or others saying, "This is who I am," or "I was born like this and I can't change." We have deemed most of these programs as normal because people around us believed they were. So, it is expected that you will follow the same programs and will live the same life as people around you, which often includes fear, insecurity, anger, guilt, and depression.

If you decide to change your life (yes, it is your decision), as hard as it may be for many people to accept, you must believe you can to start changing your life. If this feels hard at this point, it's OK; accept it and say to yourself, "I am not ready now, but I know there is a way and I will start when I am ready." Always remember, the first and most important point is not to be hard on yourself.

Be kind to yourself. You were born blessed and worthy.

Most of us were taught not to listen to our emotions but to overcome them. We were told to be strong, and that we must overcome our fears, but even if we succeed for a while, we are simply exhausting ourselves.

Your emotions are your guide to what is happening in your body. If you have positive emotions such as love, peace, acceptance, and joy, this means neurotransmitters like serotonin and dopamine are excreted in your brain, which is great for your brain and whole body. But if you have negative emotions, your body has excreted cortisol, a stress hormone, which when released, has bad implications on every cell of your body. Many people accept these emotions as normal and try to accommodate them, which can result in physical or mental disorders. Such disorders are the result of chronic negative thought patterns which have caused a change in brain and body chemistry (I discuss this in greater detail in chapter 2). Your perception of things around you and your experiences greatly impact your body. To truly unlock the potential of your mind, it's important to accept that everything you've experienced has a purpose. Most people will respond with, "Easier said than done." This is also a subconscious program that you can consciously change.

It's important to remember that severe physical or emotional trauma as a result of war or abuse, for instance, often requires professional help. The brain has an incredible ability to recover under a proper treatment plan, including pharmacological and psychological strategies.

Start by making a list of your own experience or people close to you, that seemed to not possibly have any positive outcomes but actually turned out to be in your best interest. Always remind yourself that you are one of God's best creations, born blessed and worthy, and rest in knowing this until you are ready to make this change. The effort needed from you is to make your conscious mind remember this fact and repeat it enough until your subconscious mind adopts it. Then, and only then, will these reassuring thoughts come to you automatically and become your first response during any seemingly negative situation. That said, it's important to remember it's a continuous process, so don't consider it a mission you want to get over with, falling into a same-old program.

At first, it may seem as though your subconscious mind is your enemy, but it's not. It's a powerful tool that you can use to your advantage. For example, if you take a medication and you are convinced it has a sedative effect, your subconscious mind makes sure the sedation side effect happens, even if it's a sugar pill. This is known as the placebo effect. If you feel good hearing this information, then you are ready to make the change, but in case you are not ready to accept it, remember it's OK.

Be kind to yourself. You were born blessed and worthy.

Most of us have been programmed to believe that things could not and should not be so simple, following the universal subconscious program that simple is not valuable, while effort and suffering are more appreciated. If you have decided to start this journey of well-being, give your mind a chance to breathe outside the subconscious programs it's been trapped in. Spend some time in a relaxed state, such as meditation or prayer, while taking the opportunity to identify your emotions and underlying subconscious programs. The key is to do it out of care and love for yourself, not obligation. Don't try to overthink where you got these thoughts, such as childhood experiences, news programs, or past trauma. If these thoughts don't feel right, you must work on changing them consciously. In most cases, it takes some time and just requires awareness, acceptance, and being kind to yourself. It is also expected that you will relapse back to your programmed thought pattern because like most things in our lives, time is needed to develop.

For instance, a baby needs nine months inside his mother's uterus to fully develop. Changes in a person's weight and body shape need time spent focusing on diet and perhaps dedicating time for exercise. Therefore, it is important to convince yourself that change is possible and decide to enjoy working toward it even if it takes time. Changing your thought patterns changes your brain chemistry and gene expression, ultimately changing your life.

Be kind to yourself. You were born blessed and worthy.

Accept that your emotions act as your guidance system as opposed to fighting them, and then learn how to change them. To accept that God has blessed you with this guidance system, you have to really accept that you are one of God's greatest creations, born blessed and worthy, and only from there can you find your sense of worthiness and well-being.

Below, I have listed some common emotions that may have a direct effect on your well-being.

Most Harmful Negative Emotions

- If you feel depressed most of the time and have lost interest in life, please reach out for professional help; medication may help while working on yourself.
- Guilt, insecurity, and unworthiness are also negative emotions that come from a programmed subconscious mind mostly from past childhood experiences.
- Hatred, anger, and revenge are also damaging emotions.

Most of us were raised to accept these emotions and justify them as a result of a deep program in the subconscious mind related to fear.

All of us have different subconscious programs, it is a normal part of our being. The difference lies just in which programs *you* have been exposed to. So, the first step toward your journey to well-being is accepting this, and being kind to yourself wherever you are.

Be kind to yourself. You were born blessed and worthy.

Negative Emotions

- Blame, worry, and frustration are negative emotions accepted and justified by most people as a normal response to stressful conditions.
- Boredom, pessimism, and discontentment are also negative emotions, indicating that there is an underlying thought process that needs to be worked on.

By understanding the harm you are doing to yourself, you will appreciate this emotional system as a guide toward achieving your well-being.

Positive Emotions

- Hopefulness and optimism indicate positive thought processes and the release of neurotransmitters in your brain such as serotonin and dopamine, which are great for your mood and health.
- Enthusiasm and eagerness throughout your day indicate being on the right track.
- Passion, joy, and unconditional love are the optimal positive emotions, which I wish for myself and everyone else.

It's important to emphasize that you will fluctuate between different emotions almost every day. Don't be hard on yourself. It's a continuous process; enjoy it.

One of the reasons only a few people seek professional help is the stigma attached to being a mental health patient. Some see it as a sign of weakness, but this cannot be further from the truth. Seeking guidance means you want to take control of your life, while others struggle every day. Others consider seeking professional assistance a sign of not having enough faith, which also could not be further from the truth. Having faith is believing in God's blessing, guidance and that there is a good reason behind everything. Another common reason people avoid professional help is the common belief that medication is addictive and once started, you will never stop them. This is not scientifically true as only a few psychiatry medications such as anxiolytics have an addictive potential. It is important to note that the goal of almost all treatments is not to keep you on medication forever. Most medications for neuroses are only needed for a few months, but this also depends on the patient's ability to make changes to their thought patterns.

Be kind to yourself. You were born blessed and worthy.

In my experience, guilt and fear are at the core of most negative emotions. These two feelings are, in most cases, deeply embedded in the subconscious mind during childhood from our relatives, environment, or in many cases, both. One of the first and most important things to remind yourself of in this process is to never blame others as that convinces yourself that you are a victim. Instead, accept that whatever you went through was for a good reason, and not that you deserved to experience something bad. Remember to let your emotions be your guide to what's happening inside your body, giving you clues as to whether a thought is positively or negatively affecting you. If you are overly worried about your health, for example, this is a sign that you are negatively affecting yourself, even if you think it's justified. Most people will argue this is a wise thing as you are trying to improve your health, but worrying excretes cortisol into your body adversely affecting every cell of your body.

"So what should I do? Should I not care about my health? First, I must recognize this thought doesn't feel good, so I will try to change it to a better feeling thought. I care about myself; I deserve to live a good life. I will eat the most balanced diet I can afford, do the exercise I am currently ready for, and avoid negative, stressful situations as much as possible."

How did you feel after reading these words? You must tailor them until they feel good to you. Once they feel good to you, start practicing them. First, you must believe these words by proving them to yourself from your life experiences where you felt blessed or lucky. If you feel stuck, it's OK; ask for professional help. Second, remember to repeat these encouraging words often enough until they become your automatic response. The aim is to shift toward health and well-being, not just trying to avoid illness. They might seem the same, but there are significant differences between avoiding illness and aiming toward health. When working toward your well-being, neurotransmitters such as serotonin and dopamine are being secreted, which have a good effect on your mood and health. On the other hand, in avoiding illness, you are harming yourself by releasing stress hormones that negatively affect every cell in your body.

Be kind to yourself. You were born blessed and worthy.

One more common example of fear would be worrying about your kids. This fear is accepted by most parents and justified by a deep sense of responsibility. If this worry provokes the stress response in your body and thoughts such as, "They are my responsibility. I will be blamed if anything happens to them; what am I good for if I cannot provide for my kids?", then you must admit that there is a healthier thought pattern. Most parents see their children as part of their lifetime achievement and identity. The real issue is that so many people share the same concepts resulting in the acceptance of these concepts in most communities. If you decide to change this, realizing these concepts and thoughts are stressful, spend some time reevaluating such thoughts and then change them to better-feeling thoughts. For instance: "My children are God's gift, and I trust I will be guided every step of the way in living a good life with them. I decided to enjoy every minute I spend with them." The most valuable gift you can give your children is to let them see your confidence and a deep sense of security in your daily activities, inspired by your deep knowledge of God's care and love. At that point, they will be able to live in our world knowing God is looking after them. Life is unexpected, and part of our psychological maturity is to accept this while expecting a peaceful, positive outcome.

Be kind to yourself. You were born blessed and worthy.

Guilt is one of the common negative emotions that is not only accepted but often also appreciated. Most parents make their children feel guilty about their actions with the best intention to motivate them to do the right thing. While their intentions are typically good, they induce a feeling of unworthiness in their children. Your intentions are important, but they will only be appreciated and rewarded by God . People cannot understand or appreciate your intentions and are instead only affected by how your behavior has influenced them. Knowing this should not make you feel sorry for yourself or point blame toward anyone. Fear of not being good enough also often provokes a feeling of guilt— "I am bad," or "I don't deserve anything good" —increasing the fear of not being good enough which goes on until you recognize this thought process and decide to change it. My advice is to spend as much time alone as needed in a calm place, practicing deep-breathing techniques until you are in a position where you can prove to yourself from life experiences, religion, or cultural concepts that you are blessed and worthy. You will know you are on the right track by how you feel.

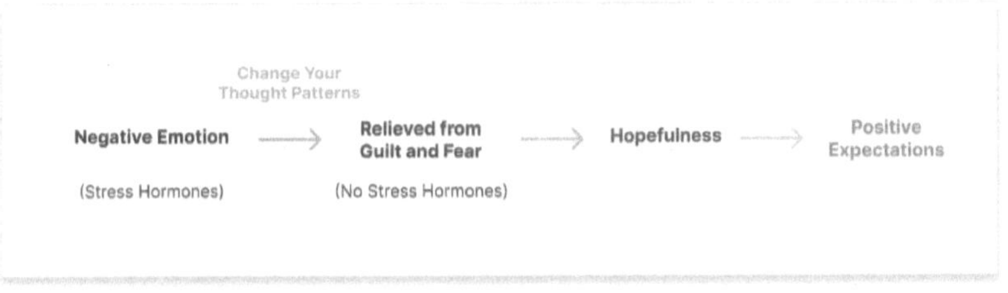

The process is not about having no problems, because our life journey is about expecting the best while working toward resolving the issues we face. It's all about your perception of what has been, what is, and what is expected. It should be a relief to know you are in control of your perception of what's happening to you. This change in pattern needs time and practice—perhaps months or even years—so enjoy knowing you are on your way and on the right path. Some will find difficulty in accepting that it might be so simple. We have been deeply programmed to accept and expect having to put in extreme effort and suffer to achieve something. As the old saying goes, "No pain, no gain," but pain means stress, and by no means can this be good for your physical and mental health.

If this is how you currently feel, that is OK, but you must aim to try to change this thought process. Any effort toward any task should be made with the intention of enjoying the process. Start enjoying every lesson, be eager, and expect the best. Such positive expectations will have positive effects on your physical and mental health. Go to the gym with the intention of enjoying the process: enjoy every minute, enjoy the positive expectation and every little achievement, and don't postpone feeling happy until you achieve your goal. The good news is that by practicing this positive expectation process, it gets easier with time. Eventually, the subconscious adopts this way of thinking and it becomes an automatic, effortless, and easy response to all your tasks.

Be kind to yourself. You were born blessed and worthy.

2

HOW STRESS AFFECTS EVERY CELL OF YOUR BODY

Stress is defined as a feeling of strain or pressure. Most consider a small amount of stress acceptable, as it may play a significant role in performance. In case you consider this true, how would you draw the line between what's normal and what's too much? Your real power lies in controlling your perception of the things around you. Stress may be related to external factors but is mainly related to your internal perception of threat.

This chapter aims to help you understand the real effect of your thoughts, perceptions, and attitude on every cell of your body. It's not only normal but expected and instinctive for every person to take care of themselves. But what most people don't realize is that their subconscious mind programs can make it difficult to recognize stress for what it really is and try to tolerate stress in a unhealthy way most of the time. Shedding some light on the biological effect of stress should be a great motive for most people to consider working on their thought processes. In this chapter, I introduce the scientific background of stress which you do not have to memorize or even understand in detail. However, knowing this information has motivated many to change their thought processes.

HPA (Hypothalamic–Pituitary–Adrenal Axis): The Main Stress Response System

Neurons are the cells of communication in the brain. The human brain contains tens of billions of neurons linked to thousands of other neurons. Thus, the brain has trillions of specialized connections called synapses. Once you consider anything stressful, this is recognized by the amygdala (the almond-shaped mass of nuclei in the temporal lobe), then HPA (hypothalamic–pituitary–adrenal axis) is activated, and cortisol is excreted. This HPA axis should only be activated in cases of real danger as part of the fight-or-flight response to save your life. Cortisol is a steroid hormone excreted from the adrenal glands. Its release is increased in reponse to stress, and feedback to the hypothalamus inhibits Corticotropin Releasing Factor (CRF) and terminates the stress response. The amygdala and hippocampus also provide input to the hypothalamus to suppress the HPA axis. High cortisol levels are toxic to neurons and contribute to atrophy in chronic stress. They eventually cause hippocampus atrophy, which inhibits the HPA axis. Atrophy leads to chronic activation of the HPA axis and increases the risk of developing psychiatric disorders (Stahl 2021, 270–71).

Like everything in our world, cortisol has two sides. It provides good functions when needed, such as in the case of low glucose levels (by increasing blood sugar) or inflammation (anti-inflammatory effect). However, if cortisol is excreted for an extended period time, it will adversely affect the immune system, bone production, and will damage the hippocampus in the brain. By understanding this stress mechanism, we can now understand the effect of stress on every cell of our body and brain. Your real power lies in your perception of what's happening around you and to you.

Many situations and thoughts that provoke fear and guilt are shared and accepted among everyone, leaving many people as victims of frustration, helplessness, and unworthiness. The reason for this is that these programs are shared on a subconscious and conscious level, giving you no real chance to evaluate and implement change. There is no room for blame in this process. If knowing this has touched something in your heart and made you feel good, this means you are ready to make the change. If not, don't be hard on yourself.

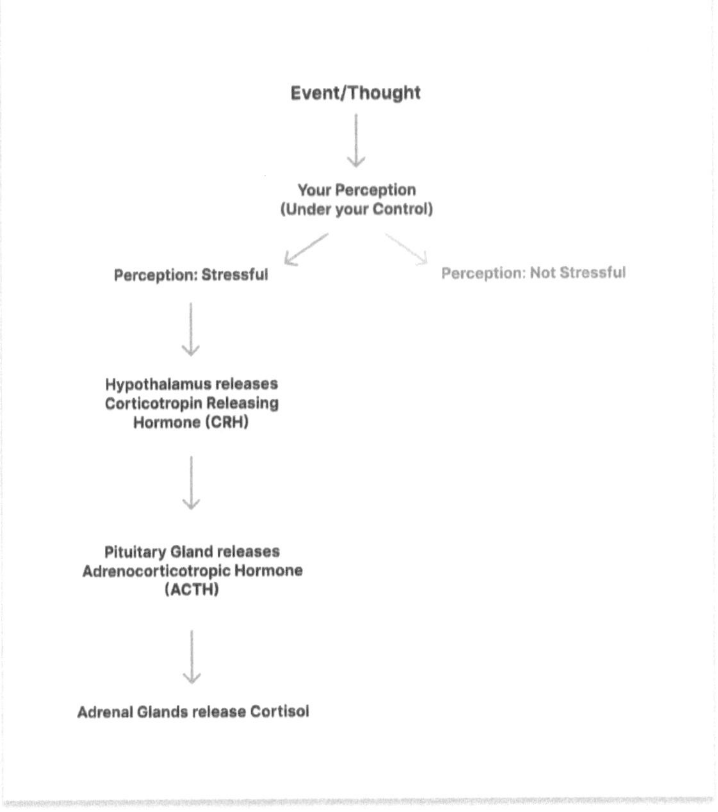

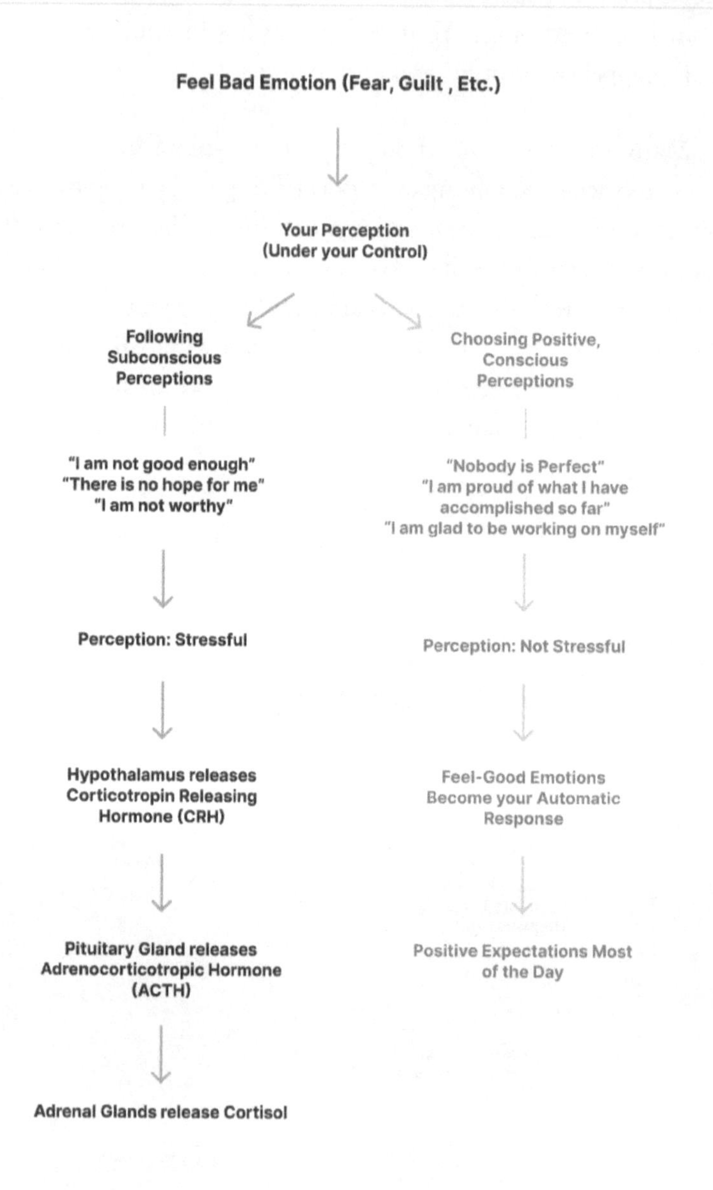

This diagram is an example that you have the power to choose how to perceive the world around you whether it be through thoughts or events.

Brain-Derived Neurotrophic Factor (BDNF)

Another important biological effect of stress is its effect on brain-derived neurotrophic factor (BDNF), which promotes the growth and development of immature neurons, enhances the survival and function of adult neurons, and helps maintain a synaptic connection. A decrease in its level will compromise the brain's ability to maintain neurons and their connections, leading to the loss of synapses or even entire neurons by apoptosis. Multiple environmental factors, including chronic stress and illness, early life adversity, and altered sleep can cause epigenetic changes that switch the genes of BDNF off and reduce its production. The decrease in BDNF may affect the brain's ability to maintain neurons and their connections (Stahl 2021, 267–68). It doesn't matter when, what, or who caused your stress, once it's recognized as stress, it will have a biological effect on your entire body. Maybe before knowing this, you felt helpless, but now you know better. Kindly allow me to remind you that the journey back to peace, love, and wellness may take some time.

Neuroinflammation

Neuroinflammation can also be a cause of neurodegeneration. Chronic stress, early life adversity, chronic sleep issues, and chronic inflammation may cause neuroinflammation. In case the microglia are activated in the brain, they release proinflammatory cytokines, attracting immune cells as monocytes and macrophages into the brain, which can disturb neurotransmission, cause oxidative stress and mitochondrial dysfunction, affect the HPA axis function, reduce the availability of neurotrophic factors, and lead to epigenetic changes, ultimately leading to synaptic loss and neuronal death (Stahl 2021, 272–73). By knowing the above information, I hope the effect of stress on your brain and whole body is clearer. The aim of sharing this information is to make you more motivated than ever to take care of your mood, thoughts, and perceptions. Knowing this shouldn't worry you, but if you are now worried, please remind yourself that all these processes can be reversed depending on your willingness to start the journey, commit to change, and asking for guidance along the way if you feel that you need it.

Epigenetics

There are more than twenty thousand genes in the human genome, but not every gene is expressed, even in the brain. Epigenetics determine whether a gene is made into specific RNA and protein or if it's ignored and silenced. What happens in your brain depends on which genes (abnormal or normal) are expressed or silenced. Neurotransmission, drugs, and environmental factors such as stress, trauma, and abuse, regulate which genes will be expressed or silenced. Depending on what stressful event happens to the neuron, previously silenced genes can become activated, and previously active genes can become silenced (Stahl 2021, 23–4). Despite there still being a lot to research and discover regarding epigenetics, you now know you are not a victim of your inherited genes.

Every day, science is proving to us how little we know about the miraculous function of our brain and body. I hope that the above information left you with a sense of pride, eagerness, and peace— proud that you are a marvelous, precious creation; eager to know more about yourself physically and psychologically; and at peace with the fact that you are under the care of a divine power, working joyfully every day toward your wellness. You may believe in this but cannot seem to benefit from it because you are trapped in so many subconscious programs that you don't get the chance to remember or apply this knowledge in your daily life, leaving you as an easy prey for your stress hormones.

By knowing this information about your brain and how it works, a deep sense of worthiness will start to develop not because of what you have done in your life, but because of who you are. When you decide to start your well-being journey, this deep sense of worthiness may be your starting point to changing your mindset. Next time you find yourself in a bad mood, don't jump to judging yourself, but give yourself a chance to remember who you really are. At that point, you will be able to look for solutions from a perspective that feels a sense of worthiness and security instead of fear and insecurity. To some, this seems like a known and simple information, not realizing the significant impact applying this mindset has on your brain and body—and by that, ultimately your whole life. You cannot control your life events, but you can control your perception of everything happening to and around you.

3
VALUABLE DISCUSSIONS FROM MY CLINIC

In this chapter, I will share some cases from my clinic that you may find helpful. It's amazing how much we all have in common, and I hope the following examples will provide insight into that. I would like to firstly discuss a case that motivated me to pursue psychiatry. It highlights the challenges faced by patients with psychiatric disorders, the stigma surrounding mental illness, and the journey to recovery from such struggles.

Once I completed my internship, I decided to spend my assignment year at a mental hospital located as close to home as possible. Honestly, I had no intention of pursuing psychiatry as a specialty at the time. Like many others, I had limited knowledge about psychiatry, as we only covered it briefly during medical school. At the time, my plan was to complete this year and then start my residency in pediatrics. One day, when I was in the clinic working alongside a psychiatry consultant, a patient came in; she was so anxious and could not stop crying. The consultant calmed her down and the patient was eventually able to explain that she had repeated thoughts that she would stab her daughter to death. She knew it was something she would never do, but could not stop the constant thought and felt helpless. I felt so bad for her and was not aware that treatment would be possible but the psychiatry consultant assured me that medication could help her. However, she then faced the stigma of seeking mental health care through her mother-in-law, who labelled this woman as crazy, asking her son to file for divorce. Despite improving and being able to take care of her family, this was not enough for the mother-in-law, who insisted her son divorce her.

Although she was still struggling with the social consequences, we were all grateful for her improvement. The only word that could begin to express how I felt was lucky. I felt lucky to be part of this patient's improvement and that was the turning point on my perspective of psychiatry.

Next, I will give you some examples of cases in my clinic that may help you understand yourself more.

Anxiety Symptoms

The foundation of anxiety is fear. As mentioned before, fear is an emotion indicating a thought pattern mainly because of subconscious programs. But which subconscious program exactly?

Many people consider fear a protective mechanism helping protect you from psychological or physical harm. On other occasions fear is considered a motivation to reach a certain goal. It's accepted by most people to worry about exams, health, deadlines, and the list goes on. Worries vary in severity, leaving many people unable to enjoy a few hours every day. When we start using our emotions as our guidance system, how do we feel when we get these thoughts? We will start to distinguish which thought is good or bad for us. I will begin by giving examples of stressful conditions you can face daily, hoping they will be a light to your journey of well-being. It is important to start understanding our emotions instead of resisting them, because when we fail to control them, we feel defeated.

If your car doesn't start in the morning, you may end up running late for work. How does this feel? Most people will be frustrated, worried, or even blame themselves or someone else. What do all these emotions have in common? Stress hormones are excreted, resulting in the stress mechanism turning on. Most people will accept this reaction and consider it normal—or even worse, beneficial to motivate or protect them from any of these events happening again. Because these reactions are often shared by so many people around us, only a few will recognize it as harmful and will try to do something to prevent this unhealthy reaction. The first and most important step is to recognize that this thought is not beneficial to accept but is detrimental. Then try to shift your perspective and find better-feeling thoughts? Feeling good means, no stress hormones, which is a huge step for many. In my practice, the best and most beneficial way to shift your perspective is to prove to yourself that everything is working out by using any personal experiences that you thought were bad, but turned out to be in your best interest. For example, you might say, "Yes, I am late for work, but maybe it's for the best." It cannot just be words because that won't be enough. We must be willing to do the work, and by work, I mean taking the time and being willing to go through life until you totally believe that everything is working out for you.

Start by making a list to remind yourself of occasions that initially seemed to only be negative but actually had positive outcomes. For example, when being late saved you from an embarrassing or even dangerous situation. Who can perceive being late as having a good reason? We are programmed to see only good or bad, so perceiving being late as a good reason is very difficult but you must remind yourself that in many cases, situations that seem bad are a good step in disguise for a great end. Consider it a process, like going to the gym, aiming to reach a specific goal. Enjoying the process is the real indicator that you are on the right track. If you are not ready, remember that feeling guilt is not in your best interest. Guilt feels bad, meaning your body and brain are under stress, so rest in the knowledge that you will start once you are ready.

Most of my patients shared fear as a common emotion, which differs in severity from one form of anxiety to another, and if not treated early enough it can develop into more serious disorders including depression. It's never too late for anyone to start changing their mindset to a healthier one; all it depends on is how much practice you will need to start your journey back to well-being.

Be kind to yourself. You were born blessed and worthy.

Diagnosed with a Medical Condition

So many of my patients came to my clinic after being diagnosed with a medical condition, referred to me by their physician, and in most cases worried about this referral. "Why did my physician refer me to you?" was a common first reaction among my patients worried about the stigma of therapy, feeling defeated, ashamed, and even angry. Who can blame them for worrying about this stigma especially if their physician did not properly explain the need for the referral.

Being diagnosed with an illness can make patients worried depending on their perception of the illness, which in most cases is related to subconscious programming shared by the community they live in. Remember, your subconscious mind is like a storage room containing all the attitudes, beliefs, and emotions you have stored without intending or even noticing. For example, if someone is diagnosed with diabetes, most will react with fear from what is considered a chronic disorder, deteriorating over time, and this can affect their entire life. Children come to me angry: "Why me? It's not fair," refusing the diet instructions, acting out, and often fitting the criteria of depression. What makes this perspective so accepted is that it will be shared by most people around the patients. They may feel sorry for them, blame them, or even ignore their pain in most cases, without intending to harm the patient. It's important to understand that people around us also respond according to their own subconscious attitudes, beliefs, and programs. By giving them the benefit of the doubt, you relieve yourself from judgment, blame, and negative behaviors that can trap you in a thought process fueling the stress mechanism. The only person you can control is yourself. If knowing this makes you feel bad, it's OK, but understand this is also a subconscious program of trying to find security by controlling the people or circumstances around you.

I have discovered that providing my patients with detailed information about their illness has been most effective. This approach helps them better understand their condition and ensures they do not feel any form of judgment. Diabetes is just like any other disease; as medical interventions advance; better treatment plans also develop. Just a change in perspective can relieve a person from the stress hormones. Many people surrounding an individual attempt to persuade them to accept their circumstances while cautioning them about any adverse effects, resulting in feelings of stress, fear, helplessness, and potential depression.

Every chance I get, I remind my physician colleagues in other medical branches not to traumatize the patient with any news of a condition without giving them enough realistic and optimistic information. Like me, most physicians don't learn enough about the patient's psychological well-being in medical school, so it varies between physicians depending on their interests or experience in this field. Although they care about the patient's well-being, not having enough information about this field makes them unaware of the psychological effects of their treatment plan and the outcome of their patient's recovery. The good news is that new studies are now being done in the medical field regarding the power of subconscious beliefs on the outcome of treatment. This was why I always took the chance to spread this message in every hospital I worked in.

Once I establish a positive relationship with my clients, I help them shift their thought patterns and provide a fresh perspective on their treatment. In the example mentioned above on the patient diagnosed with diabetes, I prioritized making them feel heard and accepted by acknowledging their concerns. I explained that there have been significant advancements in diabetes treatment and that ongoing research promises continued progress. Providing practical examples for the patient can help facilitate their understanding and acceptance of this knowledge. By helping them let go of the victim narrative, they shift to seeing this condition as a simple messenger just guiding them to their well-being. For example, now they must take care of their eating habits, which could have a great effect on their whole health, preventing a more serious disorder from evolving. By changing this perception, they move from a stressful thought process to a more eager and grateful thinking pattern where they can see this stressful condition as a chance to practice the gratitude mode. Being educated about the power of the subconscious mind and how it affects our health has helped many of my patients make this change. Some patients will need to start medication to help them with their mood while working on this change in their thought pattern, and this is totally fine.

Be kind to yourself. You were born blessed and worthy.

Diagnosed with a Life-Threatening Disorder

Stress from a life-threatening disorder likely started long before the patient received a diagnosis. Your subconscious mind is filled with fear and negative expectations unintentionally stored from what you have heard from your surrounding environment (such as family, news, or social media) regarding these disorders. In some cases such expectations arise from a personal experience or an experience gone through by someone close to you. Just by being diagnosed or still underdiagnosed, your subconscious mind will flood you with all its previously stored knowledge charged with highly intense emotions as an automatic response. We have been conditioned to fear illness, making the patient vulnerable to anxiety. This fear can directly impact the immune system, which is essential for healing; it's like destroying your own army out of fear of what you perceive as the enemy. This fear is shared by most human beings and considered a protective tool, driving them to take care of their health, eat better, and go to the gym. It's true that eating healthy and exercising is good for you, but only if you do it out of love— for your life, body, and existence. Love to be the blessed, worthy creation you are. Never do it out of fear of disease because in that case, your disguised "good intentions" are just deceiving you and actually harming your body and brain by the continuous release of stress hormones.

How do you feel when you hear about a terminal illness or a disabling neurological disorder? How you feel will depend on your subconscious programs shared by the community and culture you belong to. After being diagnosed, it is common for patients to experience a range of emotions, such as fear, guilt, helplessness, anger, and depression. These emotions trigger the release of cortisol, affecting every cell in your body, including brain cells. It is important to understand that many individuals are stuck in subconscious programming and may only view recovery as possible through a miracle. Recognizing this, and changing your mindset, can be a game-changer in the healing process.

As defined by most humans, a miracle is a surprising and welcomed event not explicable by scientific or natural laws and is considered the work of divine intervention. Most people consider miracles a rare incidence. This is a subconscious program shared amongst so many people, and as a result, they rarely expect them to occur. Is getting pregnant not a miracle? Is a seed growing into a fruit not a miracle? Is your immune system making you recover from an illness not a miracle? Is the rain not a miracle? Are you not a miracle?

We have become so used to these things happening daily that we consider them normal. Remind yourself that these are, in fact, miracles. They should not only be words; you must take time every day to prove it to yourself from your own life, a continuous practice until the subconscious mind adopts it. By reading about people with near-death experiences who recovered from these disorders, a patient can change their mindset and shift toward a more positive attitude, which will have a great effect on their recovery. Only then will the patient be relieved from the stress hormones, and the immune system can return to doing the work it was created to do.

Be kind to yourself. You were born blessed and worthy.

Fear from a Global Event, Such as a Pandemic or War

Two factors play an essential role in the stress associated with a seemingly adverse global event. First, this stress is shared among so many individuals, affecting each person and increasing concerns, anxieties, and fearful subconscious programs in one another. Such shared fear results in a snowball effect, growing with every experience or warning about these events. The second factor is feeling helpless in protecting yourself or the people you care about. Fears, worries, and depression are not only accepted but expected as a normal response by most people. Whoever can change their mindset, relieving their body and brain from the toxic effects of stress, will survive with the most minor damage possible, if any. It is totally accepted and expected that you will initially experience all kinds of emotions in a situation like this, but the aim is not to focus on your negative emotions but to find your way back to balanced, conscious thinking. Many believe that everything happens for a reason and that everything is ultimately controlled by a higher power. By asking for God's guidance, you will feel much better. It is easier for some than others, depending on their belief in a higher power, which can only be measured by the degree of relief it brings. Practicing this belief by proving it to yourself is the best and only way to change your underlying programs such that your automatic response is confidence that everything is working out for you. Dealing with stress will get easier day after day, and although it needs awareness, acceptance, and persistence, the result is guaranteed. Any change, even if minimal, will positively affect stress levels and, as a result, every cell of your body, so change is totally worth it. It took some of my patients only a few weeks and others longer to change their thought patterns. It's worth mentioning that slipping back into old thought patterns is expected, and explaining this to my patients helped them reduce their feelings of guilt, which would be a trap. Another important point I want to make is that some people feel terrible when they see someone else suffering. So, when you see someone suffering from an illness, trapped in a war, homelessness, or in any situation considered severe, most people will agree that the normal human response would be to feel empathy toward them. Anyone not sharing this feeling may feel guilty or be judged by others. If you use your emotions as a guide, you will realize that fear, guilt, hopelessness, and depression are not in your best interest. Being trapped in a negative thought pattern will help no one, but if you start changing your mindset, remind yourself that everyone is here on their own journey. Taking care of yourself physically and mentally is the best thing you can do because only then can you help others. Ask yourself how you can help without letting negative emotions drain you. A good example would be to assist someone stuck in mud; it is essential to find stable ground first. Only then can you provide effective help. Suppose you involve yourself too early in the rescue process. In that case, you risk getting dragged into the mud and endangering everyone, including yourself. Once you feel you are standing on solid ground, you can actually help others. From my experience, patients ready to change this mindset found relief from stress and started to enjoy the eagerness and joy of adopting this new thought pattern.

Be kind to yourself. You were born blessed and worthy.

Social Anxiety

Feeling anxious about being judged in social events is more common than most people realize. This fear of judgment comes from a core belief in the subconscious mind of not being good enough. Nobody was born with this belief; it is typically acquired during childhood. During these early years, you are most vulnerable. You accept whatever message you receive without questioning it, especially if charged with emotions. You store these messages in your subconscious mind and consider them true, until you recognize and change them on a conscious level. For instance, if a child gets yelled at by an angry parent, they store feelings of fear, anger, and insecurity in their subconscious. In most cases, the parent does not mean to scare the child but is displacing their anger due to marital, social, or financial stress. If you are a parent, the most important step is to accept that you did your best with the knowledge and skills you had while raising your child. I sometimes recommend that the parent admit it to the child, relieving them from guilt and rebuilding a new and healthy relationship with their child. On the other hand, I recommend the patient recognize and accept that this fear of judgment is an unhealthy subconscious program they adopted from childhood, which they were not responsible for, but can now change through awareness and acceptance. There is no room for blame. We are all humans but on different life journeys. Some people may not be ready to forgive, but at least they can accept human nature. By accepting that it is just a subconscious program, you can start your well-being journey by proving to yourself how blessed you are.

Start by writing down a list of things you are grateful for, starting with being born and having a body. You recognize your worthiness from the fact that you are one of God's best creations, and nobody can take this away from you. If you apply this to the people you feel afraid of being judged by, you will understand and accept that we all are humans on different journeys under continuous never-ending blessings from our creator. The person you are worried about being judged by, regardless of how much you worry about their judgment, is only human, has made mistakes, and has weaknesses regardless of how important this person may be. It is not uncommon for some of my patients to take medication to help control their anxiety while adopting this new thought pattern. I explain that if I must choose between them being anxious and suffering from stress hormones or on medication, I would without hesitation recommend medication.

Start by adopting new thought patterns: *It's OK to be far from perfect*, and *It's OK to make mistakes*. Accept where you are and enjoy the small changes in your thought pattern on your journey to wellness until you find the ultimate joy in unconditional love and acceptance for yourself and others. Your emotions will always guide you; learn to listen to them as they are like a light indicating if you are headed toward wellness and love or falling prey to fear and guilt. Don't fight the negative emotions; accept them for what they are and gradually change them toward what feels much better.

Be kind to yourself. You were born blessed and worthy.

Illness Anxiety

Illness anxiety is defined as a preoccupation with having or acquiring a serious illness. Somatic symptoms are not present or, if present, are only mild in intensity. Patients experience heightened anxiety about their health and become easily alarmed about their personal health status. Such anxiety can lead to excessive health-related behaviors, such as repeatedly checking their body for signs of illness or maladaptive avoidance of medical appointments and hospitals. Despite receiving proper medical reassurance, their worries about an undiagnosed disease persist. Health concerns significantly affect an individual's daily life, affecting their regular activities. These people tend to extensively research their suspected illnesses online and constantly seek reassurance from their loved ones or doctors. There is a global subconscious fear program regarding illness that makes breaking out of this cycle not an easy thing to do for most people. This concern about illness starts young from family, teachers, and the media. Most media outlets continuously warn about illnesses; even if you are not necessarily searching, advertisements will pop up in a lot of places. I encourage people to read about, research, and concentrate on health, not illness. Eat healthy food, exercise (hopefully daily), and meditate, not out of fear of illness but out of a deep gratitude for life, your body, and a sense of worthiness. Medication can help improve mood and anxiety symptoms, but changing the underlying thought pattern is the actual goal. When I start my patients on medication, I advise them to consider them a gift from God to help them start this journey as easily as possible; feeling guilty or disappointed about starting medication will not help and instead have an unwanted adverse effect.

Anxiety about the Future

Many people share the same subconscious dream of the perfect life. Most of these dreams have been shared in people's subconscious minds without choice. They have been planted in the subconscious from our culture, family, and social media (which is far from innocent). It's very healthy to have dreams and put them into reality;

this is what we were born for, but I would encourage you to evaluate these dreams on a conscious level first. You will know the difference when you start listening to your emotions. Your dream should make you feel eager, not stressed. Whenever it starts feeling stressful, reevaluate on a conscious level.

No one doesn't want to have money, a family, a healthy body, freedom, or independence, but priorities vary from one person to another. Always start with the goal that makes you happy; this indicates you are heading in the right direction. Whenever you feel stressed, reevaluate and remember that your emotions are helping you, so don't fight them; accept them and let them help direct you toward the right path.

So many people come to my clinic exhausted from their families and community, judging their achievements. Many spend most of their years, even after reaching adulthood, trying to prove themselves to a family member or even a stranger, not realizing early enough how much they are harming themselves. Most of them come not only with anxiety symptoms but with secondary depressive or medical conditions that have been complicated by the underlying anxiety symptoms, which keep them continuously under the thrall of stress hormones. In many cases, people believed this was how things were supposed to be, and they felt a sense of relief when they started to understand the underlying programs. This understanding helped them let go of guilt, fear, and feelings of unworthiness, and begin their path to wellness.

Be kind to yourself. You were born blessed and worthy.

Anxiety from Marital Conflict

I saw patients suffering from marital conflicts regularly. In most, if not all cases, they try to convince me that they are a victim of whatever abuse they describe, whether physical, emotional, or financial. Most people deeply expect that marriage is a conflictual relationship. Most patients struggled to accept my suggestion to begin working on themselves and instead sought my help to change their partner or circumstances. First, I make it clear that in cases of physical abuse, you must secure your safety. There is no way around this, and no compromises are allowed.

Only once you are safe should you start working on yourself. Many people consider a relationship as a partnership in which there is give and take. This concept sounds fair and healthy, but it leaves you in a trap of depending on your partner for your happiness and making your partner happy. This sense of responsibility and commitment makes it harder to maintain a healthy relationship. When you remind yourself that your partner is a human being with subconscious programs like you and is on their own journey, the blame, fear, and judgment begin to disappear.

I encourage partners to find their sense of security, worthiness, and self-love before depending on their partner. Only then can they experience the real meaning of sharing love. It's not about making me happy but sharing my happiness with you. You can deal with any relationship in a healthy manner by working on your subconscious programs that provoke fear and insecurity, and moving toward feeling secure and worthy.

If you really want to test your worthiness and unconditional love, imagine how you would feel if your partner left you. If you predict feeling depressed, worthless, or taken advantage of, then you have to work on this. If you predict feeling angry and frustrated but can move on, you are in a better place, but there is room for improvement.

Most people misunderstand unconditional love. They tend to share the same subconscious programs of associating it with weakness, abuse, or take it for granted. Unconditional love is actually associated with a deep sense of worthiness and is a blessing to yourself and all other humans, your partner included. With such love, there is no room for fear, as love and fear cannot occur simultaneously or in the same relationship. By loving yourself enough, reminding yourself that you were born worthy and blessed, and loving others unconditionally, you will feel secure in whatever happens in your relationships or life circumstances. The good news is that you will spread this to all the people around you, especially your children, who adopt your attitudes and beliefs on a subconscious level.

Be kind to yourself. You were born blessed and worthy.

Anxiety from Work Conflicts

Many individuals associate work with constant stress, which has become accepted as the norm. This pressure is often viewed as motivation toward achieving success. However, this stress may intensify during certain circumstances, such as working toward a specific goal or experiencing conflict. This concept has been adopted by many people's subconscious minds, which is why many don't question it. If they discuss it, they would probably get the same response as most people around them, especially someone from the same culture and mindset. The change can only begin when you start questioning these programs; only then do you start to free yourself from them. Indeed, you are not responsible for these programs, but you can change them consciously.

If you perceive your work as stressful, you are under the mercy of your stress hormones, regardless of how much you justify it. If you don't like your job and are doing it only for money, the first step is to accept where you are and enjoy whatever you can in this job. Now that you have relieved your brain and body from the side effects of the stress hormone, you can find a new thought process.

Some resistance from your conscious mind is expected when starting this change. The subconscious mind simply makes whatever programmed thought you have come easily until you question it and make the conscious changes. When you question the concept of work, money, and self-worth, try to shift to a more joyful and peaceful thought pattern. You must always start with your self-worth. As you convince yourself that you were born worthy and blessed, you can redefine what your work and career mean to you. Now, you are not on a journey to prove yourself; you are on a journey to enjoy discovering your true power and sense of worthiness. It's important to remember that simply saying something is not enough to cause change. To truly make an impact, you must repeatedly think and feel emotionally charged thoughts, which takes time and practice. Seeking success in your work for financial or self-actualization holds in its deep meaning a fear of failure on either of these dimensions. No matter how disguised or rationalized this fear is, it has the same effect of releasing stress hormones.

If you decide to pursue your career with a strong sense of purpose and feel supported every step of the way, work will no longer feel like a source of stress. However, this does not mean you won't face challenges, as they are a natural part of life. The key is how you decide to approach these challenges—with a desire to find solutions or a fear of failure. Your perception determines your level of control, so taking control of your thought patterns is essential. It's also important to note that not all subconscious programs are harmful. Once you become aware of the true potential of your mind, it's your responsibility to select the programming you wish to adopt.

Be kind to yourself. You were born blessed and worthy.

Obsessive-Compulsive Disorder

Obsessions are repetitive and persistent thoughts, images, or urges. They are intrusive and unwanted and cause marked distress or anxiety in most individuals. Compulsions are repetitive behaviors (such as hand washing) or mental acts (such as counting) that an individual feels driven to perform in response to an obsession. Compulsions are not done for pleasure, although some individuals experience relief from anxiety or distress as a result. From my clinical experience, in most cases, patients suffering from OCD have suffered for years from obsessive thoughts. But they are perceived by the patient as their own thoughts and silly, so the patient falls into the trap of feeling guilty about being unable to control it. In many cases, they spend years not talking to anyone about it, and it often takes time to open up even to their mental health professional. They frequently feel shame and guilt and describe themselves as weak.

Most OCD patients have an underlying anxiety disorder and perfectional personality traits developed from a deep subconscious program of not being good enough, leaving them prey to fear, guilt, self-doubt, and depression. Trapped in this subconscious program since childhood makes these patients vulnerable to developing anxiety and OCD disorder, which in most cases is complicated by depression. Most OCD patients have a parent with OCD traits. Being raised by such a parent increases the chances that the patient develops anxiety, OCD, or depressive symptoms. As I have previously explained, children adopt so many subconscious programs from family and culture while growing up.

My first aim is always to relieve my patient from this deep sense of guilt by making them realize the nature of the condition, which is a huge step in the patient's recovery. In most cases, we decide together that it's in their best interest to start medication considering the long journey of suffering. The second most important step is to learn not to resist the thought but instead to accept it and then replace it with another, healthier thought. Resisting it means fighting against your own mind, which already describes this obsession as silly. This increases stress levels and leaves no room for changing to another healthy thought pattern. I explain the nature of this thought-changing process and that it may need some time, which is welcomed by the patient because they have hope in the recovery and belief in the healing process.

Most patients leave the clinic from the first visit happy, relieved, and excited to enjoy their way to recovery. One of my young female patients after recovery, using both pharmacological and psychological treatments, improved to the degree that she decided to publish her own book to inspire more people. I remember the joy I felt when I first received a copy of this book. This is a real example that recovery not only affects patients but their family, friends, and in this case, many readers. Her book was written in a sincere way that I was sure it touched the heart of its readers. I have many other examples of patients who, after relief from their suffering, started sharing their experiences and healing processes with other people through different social media channels. Nothing makes me happier than seeing my patients eagerly and joyfully spreading well-being. They are living examples of humans who found their way back to wellness.

Be kind to yourself. You were born blessed and worthy.

Depressive Disorder

Depression is characterized by a depressed mood most of the day, nearly every day, markedly diminished interest or pleasure in all, or almost all, activities. Feelings of worthlessness or excessive and inappropriate guilt are also usually part of the patient's suffering. It may be surprising that some depression can occur in children and adolescents, which may be presented by irritable moods.

Let's start first with adults, it's important to note that depressive symptoms, especially if they cannot be explained by any new life events, can be caused by organic reasons such as hypothyroidism, vitamin D deficiency, and in rare cases cancer (like pancreatic cancer). If the underlying medical condition has been managed, then the depressive symptoms should improve. So medical assessment is always the first step for an appropriate diagnosis and management.

In most cases, depression is a result of chronic struggling with a subconscious program like: "I am not good enough," resulting in insecurity and guilt feelings since childhood. During childhood, children fight against these programs because they don't feel good. As a result, they exhaust their coping system, or leave their body and brain a target for cortisol and its side effects.

Adults at work may be able to achieve what most would consider success, but at what expense? All this comes back to fighting the emotions of guilt, insecurity, and worthlessness, but who could blame someone for trying to be successful? The subconscious mind feeds them continuous thoughts, giving them no chance to evaluate and consciously choose which thought pattern to adopt. Most people believe "no pain, no gain," "life is not fair," and "you are worth what you earn." You are and always will be free to adopt whatever beliefs you want. I suggest you evaluate these thought patterns and choose whatever feels good. You adopted your subconscious beliefs from other individuals without consciously choosing them which has caused you to suffer.

The media is far from innocent; how many times do you hear unhealthy messages while watching a movie or TV program? Most people are not using their conscious minds while watching, so these beliefs go directly into the subconscious mind, especially if emotionally charged, without evaluation. I don't want you to adopt any thought pattern; I want to invite you to release yourself from the subconscious programs that you are under the control of and to find your way back to your sense of worth.

In mild cases of depression, patients start blaming whoever or whatever they consider responsible, but afterward are eager to change their thought processes. In the case of most moderate or severe depressive symptoms, starting medication is in the patient's best interest. Medication at this stage is important to help with the biological changes done to the brain as a result of depression.

Regarding depression in children, it's not as common as in adults; but most patients are late to seek help. As a result of the subconscious programming that your children are your responsibility and a reflection of your success, some believe it's a personal failing if their children need help. In many cases, parents come to the clinic disappointed that their children need psychiatric consultation, even if the child is asking for an appointment .

It's worth mentioning that most people use the word *depressed* too easily, trying to express that they are not satisfied with what is going on in their lives. They don't realize that by using this word, they awaken all the subconscious programming shared by the many people from their environment or even the people they follow on social media. The subconscious will continue flooding them with these beliefs, making these beliefs seem normal and not giving their conscious mind a chance to evaluate, and as a result, expect to feel depressed daily. Remember, your subconscious mind is not your enemy; it's like a storage system that doesn't evaluate or assess the content but floods you with all the information stored, intentionally or not, when provoked by a situation. By using it to your advantage, you can program it with beliefs that are in your best interest, such as love, eagerness, worthiness, and health.

4

FOUR-STEP PRACTICE GUIDE TO WELL-BEING

I hope you have read the earlier chapters in this book before starting this practice. The book will give you some important explanations and background, so it's important to read the book carefully and repeat each part until you feel good about the information. This is an indication that your subconscious mind has adopted it as good and beneficial information for your well-being.

If some information doesn't feel good to you, don't be hard on yourself, and don't try to push yourself. Say to yourself, "It's OK where I am; it just takes time; it's a continuous process." Just by saying this repeatedly, you have avoided being pressured or stressed. Remember, fear is just an emotion. Most got used to it as a defense mechanism under the impression that it's protecting them. Understand the fear, and don't try to resist or blame yourself for still being in this thought pattern.

If you are not ready, that's totally OK. Only start when you are ready.

This practice is for those who may be struggling with their daily lives and not feeling their true worth, joy, love, and happiness that they were meant to experience. If you are experiencing significant suffering and feeling desperate, I strongly recommend seeking the help of a psychiatrist. A mental-health professional will have many treatment strategies available to help you begin your journey toward wellness.

The key to success in this practice is to feel good while doing every step and to have the commitment to put in the effort out of love for yourself. I cannot stress enough that the process must always feel good to you. For this reason, I used very few instructions related to how and when to start this practice to avoid turning it into an obligation. Turning it into an obligation will convince your mind that there is something wrong with you, making it a process that you must finish to achieve a goal. The purpose of this practice is to remind you of who you really are, it's just that your real self is buried under several subconscious programs. You don't have to do this practice—you deserve to do it—to find your way back to the inner peace, love, and joy you deserve. It's not a practice that you have or will do for a specific time, it's a mindset shift affecting your whole life. It's an individual decision, so you cannot force anyone to join you in the process, no matter how much you love them. Still, you can be a living example of the change you wish for others.

First Step

This step is the most important as it's the starting point for your wellness. It is so simple that your programmed subconscious mind will automatically resist it as it goes against existing programs present in your mind including:

- You must continuously prove your worthiness.
- Everything needs hard work (if it's not hard it's not worthy!).

Start by dedicating ten to fifteen minutes every day for the next month on what I call your well-being time. You have to sit alone which is difficult for some people who depend on others' company. Stay as relaxed as possible, in fresh air, if possible, and drink whatever you like (e.g., coffee, juice, hot cocoa). The aim is to enjoy feeling relaxed and that you deserve to take care of yourself. The most important point in this step is not to hurry to engage in your life events.

Most people care about themselves. They care about healthy food and daily exercise but forget that mental well-being is just as important. Your mental well-being will help you make smart food choices, smart exercise choices, and smart social decisions. So, love yourself enough to start this process.

The goal is to give your mind a chance to breathe outside the programs it's trapped in to evaluate and adopt new healthy ones.

1. For ten to fifteen minutes in the morning (you should not be in a hurry), remind yourself how blessed you are. It cannot be perceived by you as an obligation; you must find joy in starting this well-being process. If you feel you must do it, you have activated a program in your subconscious mind of setting a goal and only being relieved when it's done. The goal is to embrace the belief that it is OK to be where you are currently in life. To reinforce this idea, place this phrase somewhere visible in your daily routine, such as in your car, on your computer, or as an affirmation on your phone: I am kind to myself; I was born blessed and worthy.
2. Use whatever makes you happy and enjoy light music and fresh air. If not possible, surround yourself in warm lighting and comforting smells.
3. Remind yourself you are doing this because you deserve it, not because something is wrong with you. Enjoy starting your wellness routine.

4. It's completely normal that your subconscious mind will start flooding you with all the issues you are worried about. Don't blame yourself; it's part of your mind's nature.

5. Don't try to resist these thoughts or emotions but accept them and decide to postpone dealing with them .

6. Start writing (or take mental notes) of examples from your own life to prove your worthiness to yourself. You can start by being born healthy, and by that, you are able to enjoy many things in life, like seeing, walking, playing, and thinking. What did you do to get these blessings as a baby? If you were born into a nice, warm family, what did you do to deserve to have this? What did you do to deserve to be alive? Do this until you prove to yourself that you were given so many good things that you took for granted. Everyone is on a special life journey that includes some difficulties, and no one is an exception. You are alone, so you don't need to justify, pretend, or worry about any judgment.

7. The key is to enjoy this process and remember to listen to your emotions. If any step doesn't feel good, there is an underlying thought that needs to be addressed. In most cases, this thought is related to subconscious programming that you were not responsible for but certainly able to change once you become aware of them.

8. If you try for a few weeks with no obvious improvement, you can seek professional help. Some people feel safer under professional care.

The aim of this step is that you

1. Remember you are important.
2. Understand your emotions, do not try to resist them.
3. Be kind to yourself.
4. Start realizing your worthiness, which will reflect on your realization of the worthiness of all around you.

5. Repeat this process for however long it takes (usually weeks) until you really believe in your worthiness.
6. Don't jump too early to the second step. Your subconscious will encourage you to do so, from a place of achievement. Remember, the aim of this step is to relax in knowing and enjoy the process.
7. Don't share your progress with anyone who didn't already start working on their thought process. It's an individual journey, and not everyone is ready at the same time.

Common expected traps in this step:

1. It's too simple to be true. If it were so true, why don't all people know it or do it?
2. These are just words. How can words change my biology?
3. I am not a weak person, and I can master anything.
4. Admitting I need to change means I am a patient and need psychiatric help.

I need to remind you not to resist any negative thoughts; they are just subconscious programs. When you accept them as part of mental and spiritual life development, you take away their power. Resisting them gives them more power. Acceptance with no blame and gradually changing to a healthy mindset is the key.

Step 2

I cannot remind you enough not to jump too fast to the second step. Practice feeling born blessed and worthy until it's your automatic response while living happy events, such as enjoying your success or in the case of a challenge, when you find eagerness in searching for the solution, not feeling stressed and worried about it.

Knowing we live in a world of duality makes you expect good and bad things, such as day and night, health and illness, and rich and poor, but not being afraid of one over the other. Now you start to practice your belief in a higher power that will always look after you every moment of every day.

We want to start to recognize how many blessings are pointing to us. Divine love and care are the only ways to understand the unnecessity of fear.

- Is the sky itself not a miracle, with the sun coming out every day for you—yes, for you?
- Are day and night not a miracle, giving you time to rest at night and enjoy life during the day?
- You don't have to study medicine to understand that your body is a miracle. Is seeing, hearing, and eating not a miracle? Recovery from a common cold, inflammation, and bleeding, which happen every day, is a miracle.
- Is having a child not a miracle? It occurs so frequently it's considered normal, and only in cases of difficulty in conceiving or during childbirth is it called a miracle.
- These should not only be words. Take the time every day to prove it to yourself from your own life and those around you, as a continuous daily practice until the subconscious mind adopts it. The time to achieve this change varies from one person to another, so be kind to yourself in the process.

Now you will start considering quick recovery from your illness, finding love and abundance as miracles. You were born blessed and worthy, no exceptions, so start finding your way back to believing it. It's also important to remember that you may feel guilty or unworthy during this practice; accept these feelings as a normal step in the change. These feelings result from the subconscious programming that you were probably not responsible for but are now capable of changing consciously.

Some common mind traps to watch out for:

1. If I am so precious, why am I suffering?
2. I *must* prove my worthiness.

These are just a few examples of subconscious programs we adopt and suffer their consequences until we become consciously aware and start to change them. These programs leave you prey for fear and guilt, which will lead to behaviors that ensure the continuity of a stressful and depressive life. Don't try to analyze how you got these programs, as this is a waste of time and effort. Just forgive and move on, not from a point of weakness but from feeling lucky and blessed that you are now back on your way to your well-being.

Step 3

The third step would be to accept yourself for who you are and what you went through. By practicing being born worthy and proving to yourself from your own life experiences how things were working in your best interest, you will start feeling much better.

In most cases, a guilty feeling emerges regarding things you did in your life. How can feeling born worthy and doing things you consider bad go together? We have been programmed to feel guilt by our family, culture, and religion since we were children. In most cases, it was with the best intention to make you a better person and build a better community. What I want you to understand is it does not matter why you feel guilty. I want you to realize that we are all humans, born worthy and blessed, all born with different challenges; the person you consider healthy, wealthy, successful, famous, and good-looking may be suffering from the same or even worse sense of guilt and depression. Your job is to prove to yourself from your own life or even from stories of people you follow that everyone is living their own journey with challenges and blessings. This step aims to accept that you and everyone else were born blessed and worthy in this world of duality where challenges exist and to try to expect them as a normal part of life.

By changing your mindset from feeling unworthy for being born poor, suffering from a disease, in bad social circumstances, or feeling guilty and not deserving of any of God's blessings for something you did wrong, you can return to knowing that you are a worthy human being finding your way to believing your worthiness.

Start writing a list of all the things in which you consider yourself guilty. Then forgive yourself for whatever you did by knowing we are all human and that you did what you did with the best you knew how at that point, but now you know better. You don't have to show this list to anyone. Just practice this concept until it makes you feel relieved. You will start to accept that every human being on earth is born worthy and blessed with different challenges, mistakes, and regrets. You will never accept yourself totally until you have practiced giving people around you the benefit of the doubt. Don't start with the people you consider the worst or those you feel did you the most harm. Start with people you only dislike for a certain attitude, and practice giving them the benefit of the doubt.

I advise you to make two lists that you fill every day with at least one story. The first list is of situations in your past that you felt guilty about. Remind yourself, "I am a blessed human being. I did my best with what I knew then, and now I am happily moving toward the well-being I deserve." The second list would be about anyone you felt did anything wrong to you and try to give this person the benefit of the doubt. "This person is just a blessed human being like me, and their actions are the result of programming and life events. I am grateful for being guided to my well-being and wish it for everyone else."

It's also important to know that your attitude toward this person is not hoping to change their behavior. This is not your journey, it is theirs. You also don't have to invest in this relationship, but only now are you free from the negative impact of feeling like a victim.

Step 4

I believe this last step is the hardest for most people.

We were all raised believing in love being conditional, with no exceptions. Most children were raised to believe that doing good things makes your parents love you more. When you do anything they consider bad, they get angry, and they do this with the best intention to help their child be a responsible human being and do good in this world. No one can deny these are good intentions, but what do they really do to the child? They make the child not expecting unconditional love and, by natural consequence, unable to be unconditional in their life. This is the seed of fear that continues growing and affecting our lives in all ways, disguised to protect ourselves and the people we love.

It is totally acceptable for this concept to feel strange as it is against what most of us were raised to believe. The first step would be to go back to step one where you remind yourself that you were born worthy and blessed without having done anything to deserve it. It always helped my patients when I raised this and asked them to prove it to themselves from their life experiences. Then start to remind yourself that everyone you know was also born blessed and worthy. Everyone was born blessed and was faced with different challenges that shaped their life experiences. We are and will always be human beings. Repeating this every morning is the best way to start your day.

Try not to judge yourself when you do something wrong. Instead, tell yourself, "I am human and make mistakes; next time I will know better and move on with my day." During the day, try to go out of your normal routine and do something nice for someone. Feel proud of yourself, remind yourself that doing good things is also part of being human. After practicing this for a few weeks, you will be able to love people unconditionally. Unconditional love is what I hope for myself and everyone else, with no exceptions. Unconditional love is also the remedy for fear, as you don't judge people in your life and don't put high expectations on people's behaviors. Now there is no room for judgment on yourself or others, and you live life with much less fear. Less fear means less stress, and by that, more well-being is expected.

Being unconditional in your love does not mean you must accept or tolerate any behavior. It doesn't mean you have to keep a relationship with someone you don't feel like having a relationship with. Your well-being should always be your priority. You should only keep a good heart toward this person if you decide to stay in a relationship or move peacefully in different ways. What would help a lot is to remind yourself as much as you can how blessed you are that you were inspired to start this journey of well-being. So many around you are still dealing with life challenges in the same old way, which is the guaranteed way to suffer from anxiety and possibly depression.

Love Message

I hope you found this book useful. I wrote it as concisely as possible, as I want you to read it as many times as you can until you find a change in how you feel most of the day. This will be a reflection of your change in mindset.

I totally believe in your well-being, not for anything you have done but for who you really are.

In my practice, many of my patients turned their lives around, and so can you. Each one of us was born under different circumstances with different challenges. You may start your journey to well-being whenever you are ready.

Life is unexpected, and you won't be able to control what happens to you in the future, but you can control your perception of what is happening to you or around you.

The remedy for fear and guilt, the most significant emotions controlling you, is to start working on yourself to be unconditional in your love for yourself and others. It's a long process in most cases, but you will feel the change; enjoy it.

May this book guide you to love, peace, and joy wherever you are.

BIBLIOGRAPHY

Stahl, Stephen M. *Stahl Essential Psychopharmacology: Neuroscientific Basis and Practical Applications,* 5th edition. Cambridge, UK: Cambridge University Press 2021.

www.ingramcontent.com/pod-product-compliance
Lightning Source LLC
Chambersburg PA
CBHW031427250726
48656CB00002B/872